KETOGENIC DIET BENEFITS, PITFALLS AND SUCCESS

MY 6 MONTHS RESEARCH AND FINDINGS WITH 5 OVERWEIGHT PEOPLE ON KETOGENIC DIET

BY

JENNIFER ROBSON

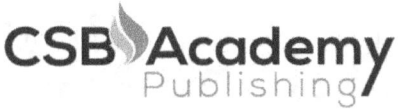

Ketogenic Diet Benefits, Pitfalls and Success

Copyright (C) 2015 CSB Academy Publishing Co.

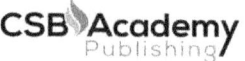

CSB Academy Publishing Company.
P. O. Box 966
Semmes, Alabama 36575, USA

Cover designed by
David Miller

First Edition

Table of Contents

A big Thank you for buying my book, I appreciate it. I am not a writer but wanted to share some of my knowledge with everyone.

If you like my work, please give me a review on Amazon.

Thanks again!

Jennifer Robson

INTRODUCTION

Everyone aims for a six pack or a lean body to look attractive, and weight conscious people are healthier too. Extra fat does not look good on anyone and has adverse effects on health, overall well-being of a person not to mention the self-confidence. Weight gain can often cause depression.

When you gain weight and become conscious of the fact that you need to lose it to become lean again, you start looking towards the different kinds of diets and exercise regimens. Some of these have been around for some years now while others come and go with the season.

This book talks about a popular low carb diet – the ketogenic diet – popular with people who feel low carb diets are effective. This is part of a three series book, which cover different diets. However, what's different about this book (and others) is the fact that I am presenting to you my research findings complete with the framework I built on the ketogenic diet – essentially an objective review of the diet based upon authenticated scientific research.

I am an independent professional researcher with a keen interest in diet regimens and health routines. I have a Master's degree in statistics, and I have worked as a freelancer for several for-profit and nonprofit organizations on various case studies and researches. This book is based on one of the researches I carried out for a company and is part of a three series book in which I will be covering my research on three popular diet regiments- the Ketogenic diet, Mediterranean diet, and Paleo diet. When I carried out this research, I wasn't allowed to publish or share my findings, as per contract, for 12 months. Now that, that period has passed, I am excited at the prospect of finally being able to share my test research along with results.

I feel that, too often, people are misled by fad diets, and when they don't experience any concrete results, they give up. Sometimes, they give up too soon, even before a diet can cause any positive changes to the body. I also observed that low carb diets are usually attacked by the media and foodies, trashing it and labeling it to be harmful for the human body. To unearth the truth, I set out to do my own research using my knowledge of research and statistical analysis, and what I found throughout this journey was amazing!

I am all set to debunk the myths surrounding the ketogenic diet because I want to help those who are looking for a concrete method to lose weight. I want to prove to you how the ketogenic diet can help you by showing you my research results. What I have discovered is that all these three diets can actually help you to lose weight and make your body lean again!

Are you ready to find out the truth of the ketogenic diet?

Let's get started...

CHAPTER 1: WHAT IS "KETOSIS" AND THE KETOGENIC DIET

The ketogenic diet is based on the process of Ketosis, so let's start with understanding what it is in essence. Ketosis simply refers to the metabolic state in which the ketone body levels in the blood reach higher than normal levels. In this state, the lipid energy metabolism is intact, leading the body to break down its own fat to provide energy to the body and facilitate everyday functions. Other names by which this diet is known include "low carb high fat diet" or "low carb diet".

We all know the source of energy for our body is glucose. Glucose comes from carbohydrates, which is present in our daily diets in starchy foods such as pasta and bread. The body breaks it down to fuel it or store it in the liver or muscles in the form of a chemical known as glycogen. In case of shortage of glucose in the body, the alternative method to acquire energy is to break down excess fat to provide a source of glucose. Ketones are a by-product of this process.

Ketones are acids that appear in the urine and build up in our blood. The presence of ketones in small amount indicates that the body is breaking down fat, but higher amounts of ketones can poison the body, which leads to a process known as ketoacidosis. High ketones level can cause dehydration and affect the chemical balance of the blood.

In simple words, ketosis is the metabolic process in which the body converts fat that can be used to produce energy because of glucose shortage, and in turn, it makes ketones. When you're eating a well-balanced diet and are healthy, the body controls how much fat it burns, and the production of ketones isn't a normal thing. However, cutting back on calories or carbs triggers ketosis. It can also be triggered after a lengthy exercise period or during pregnancy. In people who suffer from uncontrolled diabetes, ketosis indicates the inadequate use of insulin.

The Role of Ketosis

Now that you understand the process of ketosis, you might be wondering what it has to do with our body function? How is it relevant and how it helps us to lose weight through the ketogenic diet. I'll shed light on the ketogenic diet as we proceed, but first, let's see the role of ketosis.

Ketosis allows our body to function physically and mentally without carbohydrates or in its absence. When our body is deprived of calories, it is through the process of ketosis that we are able to survive. That is one of the reasons that ketosis or the ketogenic diet come under flare, because of its association with "starvation".

Ketosis and Fat Loss

Ketosis affects the blood sugar regulation positively. Sugar becomes toxic above certain intake levels or when consumed excessively. In a typical person, excess sugar is converted into fat and stored which is what makes you fat. In a person who's avoiding carbohydrates, consuming moderate levels of protein and adequate fats they may have very balanced blood sugar levels provided they eat quality veggies, fat and protein that contain the micronutrients needed in the right amount i.e., adequate caloric intake.

This model of high fat, moderate protein and low carbohydrate intake provokes ketosis. In the absence of glucose, the main concern of the body is to create ketones for the fuel, which essentially means burning fat and this is done in a better way than simply restricting your calories like most people tend to do when they want to lose weight.

Ketosis and Satiety

A person can adapt their body to burn fat in this way, using the process of ketosis, but many view it as dangerous or difficult. Our bodies are programmed to rely on one source of fuel for years, which is through the intake of too much glucose. When you reduce or remove that glucose intake from a sugar adapted person what happens is that initially it creates high levels of disgust in them. No one can adapt to a sugar-free lifestyle overnight and for some people it can take months. This is due to the fact that even our body cells aren't used to using the alternative method to produce energy and are inefficient at using the excess fat for fuel.

Once you have passed this period, you can become what is essentially called "keto-adapted." In this state, your body has become efficient at using fat to fuel it and has essentially switched to the alternative method of producing energy.

Using glucose as the source of energy requires rapid replacement and ready availability of it in our body to be converted. When our body doesn't use glucose anymore but instead uses fat to produce the energy, then we have achieved a satiation state and reduced hunger. Our constant need to have more food and snacks is reduced, and there will not be any decrease in blood sugar levels or cognitive function if you don't eat.

Ketosis and Disease Treatment

Along with or apart from burning fat, ketosis may also be beneficial to maintain overall health and treat diseases. There has been a lot of research done in the area of starving cancer cells and ketosis. Most cancers feed on glucose and when it is no longer available studies have shown that cancer cells cannot feed on ketones for fuel and thus starve. Normal cells, however, continue to derive their fuel from ketones. Ketogenic diets are also being tested in diabetes treatment. Type 1 and 2 diabetics have responded well to the ketosis state. Other health conditions that ketogenic diets have shown positive results for include Alzheimer's Disease, Parkinson's Disease and Epilepsy. This is due to the neuroprotective nature of ketosis and its positive effects on inflammation.

Ketosis and Improved Focus

Too much glucose is one of the causes of reduced brain function and less focus leading to issues such as migraines, ALS, dementia, seizures and bipolar. Reducing the intake of glucose and making the body rely on ketones for fuel levels out its effects. All his also affects how you focus, recall information and think because ketosis improves brain function through clean fuel production.

When the body uses glucose, it produces ATP that fuels the mitochondria of the cells which acts as its workhorses. The ATP produces from glucose also produces free radicals as a byproduct that cause damage to cells and disease eventually. When the ATP is produced through ketones it is much cleaner, and the free radicals produced from it are in a lower quantity.

The Ketogenic Diet

Now that we have covered the fundamentals of the process of ketosis let's move onto the diet itself, the process being what the ketogenic diet is based on. It restricts your carbs intake to 50 grams per day and helps a person get lean in no time. This is achieved through the process of pushing the body to use fat as the primary fuel source instead of carbs.

This diet was first introduced by Dr, Hnery Rawle Geyelin in 1921 as a treatment of epileptic seizures at American Medical association's annual meeting. It is called the "new Atkins" because of its popularity among the majority of the people. This diet is high in fats, low in protein and carbohydrates and to benefit from it substantially it is recommended that the diet is well regulated by a health professional.

History of the Ketogenic Diet

The ketogenic diet has evolved since its inception as a popular way to treat epilepsy and obesity. The ketogenic diet is very much similar to fasting as both diets have more or less the same metabolic process. The similarities between the two metabolic states led o development of the diet over the years when other scientists started to study its effects and health benefits. The diet mimics the effects of fasting during food consumption.

Treatment of epilepsy

The ketogenic diet has been used to treat various clinical conditions, prime among which is childhood epilepsy. Evidence from the middle ages suggests the use of fasting to treat seizures. The use of total fasting has also emerged from the 1900s as a method to control seizures. Fasting, however, is not a sustainable method for the treatment of seizures as it cannot be undertaken indefinitely.

Due to the limitations posed by fasting researchers looked into mimicking the effects of fasting for controlling seizures and developed the first ketogenic diet in 1921. During the 30s, 40s, and 50s the diet was forgotten by the emergence of new epilepsy drugs and all but disappeared during this time. The difficult off administering the diet was another reason of its disappearance and other variations of this diet were also tried such as the Medium Chain Triglyceride diet, but they all fell into insignificance.

In 1994, a 2-year-old boy suffering from seizures could not controlled through epilepsy medications or other treatments even brain surgery, which led to the rediscovery of the ketogenic diet. As long as the boy remained on the diet, his seizures remained under control, which led his father to open the Charlie Foundation and publish a book on the ketogenic diet. Today, the diet has gained much popularity for its reasons to reduce weight.

Obesity

Complete starvation to lose weight comes with several problems, foremost among which is that it loses a lot of body proteins from the muscle tissue. As starvation continues, the loss of proteins decreases quickly but the loss of significant amount of water and muscle, up to one-half of the total weight lost is alarming and unacceptable. The ketogenic diet has been widely used to reduce weight.

An alternative approach to starvation to reduce obesity was developed in the early 70s called as the protein sparing modified fast. It provided high-quality protein, which would prevent muscle loss without disturbing the effects of starvation ketosis that were beneficial to the body such as appetite suppression and reliance on body fat and ketones for fuel.

During the same period, researchers argued and suggested introducing low carb diets to treat obesity based on the fact that it promoted less caloric intake, thus promoting weight loss. Carbohydrate levels were restricted to 50 grams or less a day in these diets.

"Dr. Atkins Diet Revolution" in the early 1970s, generated both good and bad interest in the diet, causing the largest awareness towards the ketogenic diet. He suggested a diet, which was limited only in carbohydrates, and not protein and fat, suggesting it would lead to rapid and easy weight loss, which would come without staying hungry. He provided enough research to prove his point and put forth a convincing argument, but much of his research was found to be full of methodological flaws.

Ketogenic diets and athletes

In the early years of bodybuilding, low carb diets were quite common. As the emphasis shifted to carbohydrate based diets, the low carb or ketogenic diets fell into disfavor by the athletes. Modified Ketogenic diets have been introduced for athletes and specifically bodybuilders, such as the anabolic diet and body opus. In the 80s, two more diets were introduced for fat loss, the rebound diet for muscle gain and its modified version the ultimate diet which was aimed at fat loss. The diets were difficult to implement and failed to attract much attention from the bodybuilders.

The 1990s saw the introduction of the anabolic diet by a renowned expert on the use of drugs in sports Dr. Mauro DiPasquale. The diet consisted of alternate days (5-6) of low carbohydrates, moderate protein, and high fats along with the remaining days in which you can consume unlimited carbohydrates. The premise for the diet was the low carb period during which the body would be put into the metabolic shift and use fat to produce energy. During the two days, the high carb consumption would refill the carbohydrates in muscles and promote growth. However, with insufficient backing and ambiguous conclusions, it wasn't adopted by the bodybuilding community.

The other diet, which was accepted to some degree but still lacked scientific evidence, was introduced by Dan Duchaine, a bodybuilding expert. His book "Underground Bodyupus: Militant Weight Loss and Recomposition" presented three different diets and explored many topics related to fat loss. It also gave specific food recommendation in terms of quantity as well as quality and workout recommendations but left many questions unanswered again.

CHAPTER 2: BASICS OF KETOGENIC DIET

The ketogenic diet involves eating fewer carbs, and when you eat a diet or foods that are low in carbs, it puts the body into the ketosis state. The body is able to survive on the low intake of food in this state because it switches to deriving its energy source from excess fat, producing ketones in the process.

When we allow our bodies, which is the normal case, to break down glucose for energy and consume carbohydrates it produces insulin, which stores it away as triglycerides. Insulin causes fat absorption as well as prevents the body from using it for energy. If you want to allow your body to burn fat for energy production, you will have to keep your insulin levels low and prevent them from spiking, as that's the only way the body will break down triglycerides into fatty acids and use them as energy.

Low GI and low carbohydrates are effective in the ketogenic diet because they eliminate carbs that cause insulin spikes. What the ketogenic diet does is simply not just keeping insulin controlled by consuming fewer carbs but it also teaches the body to rely more on fats for energy by increasing the fat content in your diet. By staying on a ketogenic diet, your liver learns to enter ketosis and break down fat, producing ketones to use as energy.

You can measure the amount of fat being burned during the diet using Ketostix and monitoring the output of acetoacetate.

How is the ketogenic diet different from other low carb diets?

The ketogenic diet is different in many ways than your regular low carb diet, and one of the main differences is the amount of carbohydrate and protein that you consume on this diet on a daily basis. On a ketogenic diet, your carbohydrate intake is limited to between 20-60 grams per day which means you have to keep track of the carbohydrates you are consuming daily. Your protein intake requirement depends on your height, gender and the amount of exercise that you do and it should be at a moderate level. so essentially, it is different for different people. the calories are balances from fats. When you accomplish this ratio of carbohydrates, fats and proteins your body goes into ketosis achieving the main objective of the ketogenic diet.

The amount of nutrients you thus receive on a ketogenic diet is divided between the three sources. Approximately 70 percent of calories are received from the fats consumed, 2o percent from protein and 10 percent from carbohydrates.

The important thing to remember for a ketogenic diet is that you are **swapping your carbohydrates with higher fats and moderate protein intake**. Let's see why:

How does consuming high fat and moderate protein help your body to lose weight?

In large quantities, proteins affect your blood sugar and insulin levels while fats have no effect on either. Consuming more than 2 grams/ kg lean body mass of protein can cause your blood insulin to spike for the short term. In that state, your body's ability to burn the fatty acids and provide for energy is reduced. This effect may be greater in some people than in others, and it depends on two factors: insulin resistance and exercise.

When you start adjusting your diet according to the ketogenic diet plan, you will be altering your protein, fat, and carbohydrates intake levels. Let's delve into the implications of this and take a closer look at all this entails:

Carbohydrates

The ketogenic diet largely depends on the intake of your carbohydrates along with your own metabolism rate and activity level. Consuming 50-60 grams or less of carbohydrates each day is considered as the bare minimum when following the ketogenic diet. However, if someone has a high metabolism, they may be consuming a 100 grams of carbohydrate in a day and still remain on ketosis. Similarly, if someone has diabetes, they may have to limit their carbohydrate intake to less than 30 grams to be able to achieve a state of ketosis.

Protein

In the initial stages of a ketogenic diet, the amount of protein that people consume isn't as important as it becomes in the later stages. Initially, someone may consume high amounts of protein and stay in a state of ketosis, but as the body gets better at converting the protein into glucose, you may have to limit and monitor your protein intake. Too much protein at that stage may throw a person off the ketosis state, and adjustments may be necessary.

Fat

In a ketogenic diet, the larger portion of calories comes from the fat intake, and the amount of fat that you need on a daily basis is determined after you have evaluated your protein and carbohydrate intake for each day, how many calories used during the day, and whether any weight loss is achieved. After taking all these factors into account, almost 60-80 percent of calories come from fats. This makes calorie counting essential in the ketogenic diet.

What types of fats to consume?

When consuming fats in such a large quantity, the types of fats that you consume become important. One of the researchers of the ketogenic diet who has been studying it since the 1980s warns against using oils high in polyunsaturated omega 6 fats, which include cottonseed, corn, soy, mayonnaise, and salad dressings which limit the progress of anyone trying to achieve weight loss through the ketogenic diet plan. In large amounts, Omega 6 fats can be inflammatory.

Fats that are encouraged on the ketogenic diet include those which are high in medium chain triglycerides, such as MCT oil and coconut oil. These fats are converted into ketones easily by the body. Other kinds of fats such as monounsaturated or saturated fats are also commonly consumed on the ketogenic diet such as olive oil, avocado, butter, or cheeses including the sunflower or safflower oil, which are high oleic types of oil and may reflect good choices on this diet. All these fats are high in monounsaturated fats while being low in polyunsaturates.

What does keto adapted mean for you?

It takes the body several weeks to switch to a state where it starts using fats to produce energy. However, this switch may come with some form of minor health implications because the body is getting used to deriving energy from another source, which previously it only stored. This process is called keto-adaptation, which refers to the body's ability to adapt using ketones for energy production. All persons following the ketogenic diet experience different conditions in which their body is responding to the adaptation phase.

Some people feel fatigued and sluggish when they start following the ketogenic diet, which is common and felt by most people. It may become tough doing your workouts in the same way as you adjust your lifestyle to a low carb diet. The sluggish response is caused by the switch from a high carb diet to a high fat diet but once your body has adapted to the new diet, the energy levels return to normal allowing you to feel the same as you felt on a high carb diet.

Your body's response to the keto-adaptation depends on how well you have formulated your diet plan and how well maintained it is. In particular, your calorie intake is of utmost importance here which can also help reduce the initial symptoms of adaptation. The initial symptoms of a headache, nausea, and lethargy can be reduced through sodium intake, which is often an overlooked component of the diet. Sufficient intake of sodium can help relieve these initial feelings

There is a popular belief that certain systems of our belief only use carbohydrates for energy. However, it is important to mention that it's not true, and many of our major organs, including the brain, adapt quite well to using ketones for energy, provided that the diet is well formulated and followed correctly.

While on a ketogenic diet, the body may also undergo other metabolic changes because of the drastic changes in the diet. These metabolic changes may lead to a decrease in resting blood glucose, enhancement of insulin sensitivity, lowered triglycerides and increased HDL levels which are all beneficial to maintain good heart health.

CHAPTER 3: BENEFITS OF THE KETOGENIC DIET

Low carb diets are usually under attack because people believe that the high amount of fats that they have to consume to follow this diet and achieve ketosis will lead to all kinds of health problems. Whats contrary to this and important to understand, and which most of us still remain unaware of is that, there are both good and bad fats, and while our nutrient intake is being suppressed through one source it is being compensated through another so essentially, it should create a balance of calories. Although there has been less research n low car diets, whatever research has been conducted indicated that low carbs diets have remained ahead of other diets in comparison. Let's look at the benefits of a ketogenic diet:

9 Key Benefits of Ketogenic Diet:

1. It reduces appetite

People with a good appetite always tend to consume more food than needed. One of the worst side effects of dieting is in fact hunger, which makes many people feel miserable and leads them to eventually give up the diet sooner than required. On a ketogenic diet, when you limit the carbs and shift focus to eating more protein and fat it reduces the amount of calorie intake. Therefore, cutting of carbs in the diet decreases the appetite, which automatically leads to eating fewer calories without even trying.

2. It leads to greater weight loss

Low-carb diets lead to faster and more effective weight loss compared to low-fat diets. The reason behind this is that when following a low carb diet, excess water from the body is gotten rid of, faster. The kidneys start getting rid of excess sodium due to lower insulin levels thus triggering rapid weight loss, which occurs in a week or two. However, it is important to note here that following a low carb diet is not a matter of a few months but it is a lifestyle change. Often times, people give up in some months after achieving some progress, and that is when the weight starts creeping back. It is important that in order to achieve positive weight loss results from this diet; it must be adapted on a long-term basis.

3. It reduces triglycerides levels

Triglycerides are fat molecules, the presence and amount of which in our blood overnight causes a risk of heart diseases. The main reasons for elevated triglycerides levels may be carbohydrates, especially fructose. When the carbs intake is reduced the level of triglycerides in the blood tend to decrease dramatically.

4. Enhances the good cholesterols

Higher levels of high-density lipoprotein (HDL) is the good kind of cholesterol that decreases the risk of heart diseases. HDL carries cholesterol to the liver, where it is either reused or excreted. HDL levels can be increased through the consumption of fats and by limiting carbs, which is essentially, what happens on a low carb diet. A strong indicator of heart diseases risks is the triglycerides: HDL ratio and a higher ratio indicates a higher risk of heart diseases.

5. Reduces insulin levels and blood sugar

Carbohydrates are broken down into simple sugars mostly known as glucose and released into our bloodstream, thus raising the blood sugar level. We all know high levels of blood sugar are dangerous. When this happens, that body responds by burning the cells or storing them through insulin. In healthy people, this insulin response is quick which keeps the blood sugar levels under control. However, many people have developed insulin resistance, which causes a problem. Insulin resistance means that the cells aren't affected by insulin, and it is thus hard for the body to control blood sugar levels. This is also what leads to type 2 diabetes in which the body is unable to produce enough insulin to keep the blood sugar levels down. Type 2 diabetes affects around 300 million people around the world.

So when your carbohydrate intake in a low carb diet is significantly reduced the need for insulin is also removed with it. The blood sugar level tends to stay low as well as insulin.

6. Reduces blood pressure

Increased blood pressure or also known as hypertension leads to many other kinds of health risks such as kidney failure, heart disease or stroke. Low carb diets have been found to be effective in keeping blood pressure levels under control.

7. It helps treat metabolic syndrome

Metabolic syndrome is a collection of symptoms, which includes elevated blood pressure, high triglycerides, low HDL levels, elevated fasting blood sugar, and abdominal obesity, which translate into increased risk of diabetes and heart diseases. The low carb diet has been found effective to improve all these symptoms drastically.

8. It helps improve LDL cholesterol

Low-density lipoprotein (LDL) is known as the bad cholesterol, and high LDL can lead to heart attack. However, not all LDL is equal, and the size of the particles plays an important role in this regard. People who have large LDL particles have a low risk of heart attack than those who have small LDL particles. Consuming low carbohydrates and high fats can help turn these particles large which limits the floating of LDL particles in the bloodstream.

9. It enhances training in athletes

The ketogenic diet also has positive effects on athletes who are undergoing training and helps them improve their exercise regimen. Muscle glycogen levels tend to decrease on a high fat diet and after a week the body becomes efficient in utilizing fat for energy, leading to less reliance on muscle glycogen. What this means for athletes is that their submaximal endurance exercise training and performance can be improved and maintained with ketogenic diets.

The ketogenic diet can also help improve body composition by decreasing body fat and increasing lean body mass. The body composition was greatly improved in athletes from a resistance training perspective when ketogenic diet was combined with a lifting program.

CHAPTER 4: PITFALLS OF KETOGENIC DIET

There has been a lot of backlash on low carb diets overall, let alone on ketogenic diets. It is often confused as a health-destroying diet by people who don't seem to know much about the body mechanism and biology and believe that the high fat component in the diet is going to lead to their destruction, thus, giving the ketogenic diet a bad name.

The fact of the matter is that whatever pitfalls the ketogenic diet may have; its benefits outweigh its pitfalls. By carrying out my own research, I managed to disassociate myself with the facts commonly presented with this diet. But before I can make you understand how this diet can actually help you lose weight, let's review some of the pitfalls and criticisms of this diet to better clear our doubts:

4 Pitfalls You need to know
Pitfall #1

The first pitfall associated with this diet, which was mentioned earlier as well is the "metabolic shift". When your body has to make a shift from using glucose as its primary energy source to using ketones to derive energy, it will take some time. This shift usually causes people to feel fatigued, lethargic, dehydration, or brain fog. Dehydration occurs because of water loss from depletion in the glycogen stores as the body moves towards building ketosis stores. However, these symptoms are normal, and there is nothing to worry about. They will usually last a week or two, and you will feel normal again once your body has adjusted to the change. Once the body has become used to the new process, it will have more energy now than previously which limits the low blood sugar crashes often experienced on a high carb diet.

Pitfall #2

The second pitfall of the ketogenic diet is the blood lipid profile that occurs due to a large amount of saturated fats in the diet. It may be hard for some people to center their diet around unsaturated fats, or they may unknowingly miss doing so, but issues related to blood lipid profile are facing much debate.

Pitfall #3

The third pitfall of this diet is the occurrence of micronutrient deficiencies which may occur due to limiting carbohydrates to less than 50 grams a day. Thiamin, calcium, folate, iron, magnesium, potassium can decrease as their intake in low carb diets becomes limited. However, this is something that you can avoid by taking high-quality multivitamins, which ensure that you get 100 percent of these vitamins in your system and do not face any adverse effects. Supplementing fiber supplement is also a good idea to ensure your systems runs smoothly.

Pitfall #4

The last pitfall associated with the ketogenic diet is that the level of ketones can get out of control, which can be troublesome for diabetics. Massive quantities of ketone production can lead to a drop in the pH level of blood creating an environment of high acidity. In non-diabetics, it is not a grave concern as ketone body production is controlled and regulated keeping the blood pH under normal limits.

CHAPTER 5: THE RESEARCH

Obesity is a serious epidemic affecting both developing and developed countries. This has led researchers to conduct many researchers on different diets and their implications to help affected men and women control their weights. The problem isn't just about obesity, but the various disease implications that it has for men and women. Obesity causes heart problems and leads to elevated blood pressure. It is one of the prime reasons for dyslipidemia, hypertension and diabetes as well as cardiovascular diseases. Over 200 million men and women in 2008 were reported to be obese. Obesity kills more people worldwide than most other fatal diseases!

These statistics pose serious challenges for the overall world population, and in this day and age, with our fast-paced lives are dependent upon ready-to-cook foods, fast foods and all other types of instant foods that we tend to rely and survive upon; health has become a victim of our own habits. Once you start gaining fat, you don't realize how overweight you might have gotten unless the damage has been done. Fat creeps up on our body like ants, invisible until you feel difficult to climb the stairs or realize your pants are getting too tight.

Among all the popular diets that there are, the low carbohydrate diets have faced people's reservation, and this is what this research is about. It was conducted a year back as a freelance assignment for a company who wanted to study the effectiveness of the diet in overweight and obese men and women. The spectacular results that were revealed by the participants following my strict ketogenic diet plan astonished me so much that I can't wait but share my research and study.

The aim of this study is to help the larger population understand how the ketogenic diet can help them lose weight. After all, the concept behind the ketogenic diet is nothing new, and it was developed a hundred years back for the treatment of epilepsy. It's one of the only treatments for it so there must be some truth to it after all. The ketogenic diet does seem contrary to human sense. How can you lose weight by increasing intake of fat? Isn't it the fat that you want to get rid of in the first place? And the first chapter explains the science behind fighting fat with fat. Now let's see what my research reveals

Participants

For the purpose of this research, I selected five obese and overweight participants and monitored them for a period of six months (24 weeks). 3 men and 2 women were selected to study the implications of the diet on both genders. All participants were monitored weekly for developments and any problems that arose during the research period. They were all given a diet plan for each day to follow along with recommended exercises to get back in shape.

Study

The participants were first all tested for their daily macros requirements which are the macronutrients- the big 3 nutrients our body relies on to keep itself functioning well and derive energy. Participants were tested for their daily intake requirements of fat, proteins, and carbs by taking into account their body mass index and body fat percentages. The carbs for all participants were kept below

20g with a net calorie intake of 1600g on average for each of the participants.

Below is a sample 7 days diet plan that was devised for participants:

	Day1	Day2	Day3	Day4	Day5	Day6	Day7
Breakfast	Sausage and spinach frittata coffee with heavy cream (2 tbsp)	Sausage and spinach frittata coffee with heavy cream (2 tbsp)	Cream cheese pancakes: 2 Cooked bacon: 2 pc Coffee with heavy cream (2 tbsp)	Sausage and spinach frittata coffee with heavy cream (2 tbsp)	Cream cheese pancakes: 2 Cooked bacon: 2 pc Coffee with heavy cream (2 tbsp)	Scrambled or fried eggs: 3 Butter: 1 tsp Cooked bacon: 2 pcs Coffee with heavy cream (2 tbsp)	Cream cheese pancakes: 2 Cooked bacon: 2 pc Coffee with heavy cream (2 tbsp)
Snack	Avocado: ½ hass	Celery: 5 sticks + almond butter: 2 tbsps	Cheese string: 2	Avocado: ½ hass	Bone broth: 1 cup	Raw almonds: 24	String cheese: 2
Lunch	Simple egg salad:1/2 cup Romaine	Chopped romaine lettuce: 2 cups Caesar	Cooked Italian sausage link: 1 Cauliflow	Chili spaghetti casserole: 1 ½ cup Tomato	Anti-Pasta salad: ½ cup Tomato	Cuban pot roast: 1 cup Chopped	Anti-Pasta Salad: ½ cup Sundried

	lettuce leaves: 4 Cooked bacon: 2 slices	salad dressing: 2 tbsp Chopped chicken: 1 cup	er gratin: ¾ cup		and feta meatballs: 4	romaine lettuce: 2 cups Sour cream: 2 tbsp Chopped cilantro: 1 tbsp Shredded cheddar cheese: ¼ cup	tomato and feta meatballs: 4
Snack	Almonds: 24	Avocado: ½ hass	Bone broth: 1 cup	Bone broth: 1 cup	Celery sticks: 5 almond butter: 2 tbsp	Bone broth: 1 cup	Bone broth: 1 cup
dinner	Cooked chicken: 6 oz Cauliflower gratin: ¾ cup Chopped romaine lettuce: 2 cups Caesar salad dressing: 2 tbsp	Cooked Italian sausage link: 1 Cooked Broccoli: 1 cup Butter: 1 tbsp Grated parmesan cheese: 2 tbsp	Spaghetti squash casserole: 1 ½ cup Raw baby spinach: 2 cups Ranch dressing: 1 tbsp	Pasta Salad: ½ cup Tomato and feta meatballs: 4 Raw baby spinach: 2 cups Italian dressing: 1 tbsp	Cuban pot roast: 1 cup Chopped romaine lettuce: 2 cups Sour cream: 2 tbsp Chopped cilantro: 1 tbsp Shredded cheddar cheese: ¼ cup	Chili spaghetti squash casserole: 1 ½ cup Raw baby spinach: 2 cups Ranch dressing: 1 tbsp	Cuban pot roast: 1 cup Chopped romaine lettuce: 2 cups Sour cream: 2 tbsp Chopped cilantro: 1 tbsp Shredded cheddar cheese: ¼ cup

Dessert	Lindt 90% chocolate : 2 squares	Lindt 90% chocolate: 2 squares	Lindt 90% chocolate : 2 squares	Lindt 90% chocolate: 2 squares	Lindt 90% chocolate: 2 squares	Lindt 90% chocolate: 2 squares	Lindt 90% chocolate: 2 squares

Calorie Count:

	Day1	Day2	Day3	Day4	Day5	Day6	Day7
Calories	1650	1636	1512	1386	1649	1604	1609
Fat	132g	126g	119g	112g	132g	122g	128g
Net carbs	14g	18.5g	18g	19.5g	18.5g	19.5g	18g
protein	88g	88g	78g	69g	81g	89g	90g

Note: each participant was compensated for the foods listed on the diet plan

Further Breakdown:

	Day1			
foods	Calories	Fat	Net carbs	protein
Sausage and spinach frittata	206	16g	1g	12g
coffee with heavy cream (2 tbsp)	120	12g	1g	0g
½ an avocado	114	11g	1g	1g
Simple egg salad:1/2 cup	166	14g	1g	10g
Romaine lettuce leaves: 4	4	0g	0g	0g
Cooked bacon slices:2	92	7g	0g	6g
Almonds: 24	166	15g	2g	6g
Cooked chicken: 6 oz	276	11g	0g	42g
Cauliflower gratin: ¾ cup	215	19g	2g	6g
Chopped romaine lettuce: 2 cups	16	0g	1g	1g
Caesar salad dressing: 2 tbsp	170	18g	2g	1g
Lindt 90% chocolate: 2 squares	105	9g	3g	3g

Results:

After strictly following the ketogenic diet, the participants each experienced weight loss. However, it was not easy to follow the diet initially for each of them as it takes time for the body to adapt to the new diet and derive its energy from another source. It was also difficult for those involved to adjust their routine to the new diet, but after seeing positive, they affirmed that they will continue adopting the ketogenic diet into their lifestyles. Here are the weight loss results of the participants:

	Participant1	Participant2	Participant3	Participant4	Participant5
Weight before the diet	266	273	249	312	324
Weight after the diet	173	188	175	229	211
Total weight loss	93	85	74	83	113

CHAPTER 6: MY FINDINGS

Everyone loves to look slim and smart or even a healthy weight according to their age and height. And it's true that a person should strive to maintain a healthy weight in order to live a healthy and fit life. We have already reflected upon the various health conditions that can afflict a person if they become obese. Even being overweight is not favorable for people. Weight plays an important role in people's lives because it is associated with a negative stigma. Although, in some cases and situations weight gain and weight loss is out of control of people because it might be due to a health condition or naturally, but in most other cases, if people are not conscious of their diet and don't eat healthy foods, it can quickly lead to weight gain and result in them facing ill-health.

A healthy weight has positive effects on the human mind and body. When you are at a healthy weight, you have fewer problems to deal with in terms of your health and you also look and feel good. The participants who were part of this research study were all over the weight limit which they originally should have maintained, so I noticed that most of them were self-conscious. The women more so than the men because it is somehow fed in our minds that women should be slim and petite. All participants for this study were between the age range of 25-35, which is the normal age when one should become conscious of their health and lifestyle. The men seemed to care less about their weight but as they started to feel the difference, they started feeling good as well. I think men are also conscious of what they are putting in their stomachs, but more often people tend to overcome the guilt of bad eating by overeating. The more yummy stuff, which you feel is yummy but which is actually destroying your health, you put in your stomach the more you think that it's benefitting you. That's the kind of tricks our mind plays on us when we are indulging in the high carb, high-fat foods.

However, as I mentioned earlier, the participants faced some challenges initially when they started following the ketogenic diet plan and strictly following it for a period of 6 months was tough. I'm glad that all of them managed to pull through with some encouragement and luck. Always remember your end goal when following a diet plan and if possible include other people from your friends or family with you on the diet for moral support. That is what one of the participants did to motivate himself to keep following the diet for six months. He made his wife who was more or less the same weight as him to follow the diet at home, which helped him in preparation of the foods as well as give him the moral support that you need. When you see other people around you indulging their sweet tooth, it can become hard to refrain from the temptations screaming at you. All participants did face some common symptoms of switching to the new ketogenic diet and triggering the alternative energy process in their body. Some of the symptoms reported by participants included:

Symptoms and Side Effects

Frequent Urination

When you switch to the new diet and make the body shift from the glucose-based energy system to the ketones based energy system, then after a day or two, you will start experiencing frequent urination. This is due to the fact that the body will be getting rid of the glycogen stored in the liver and muscles. Breaking these glycogen releases water so it's important to drink more water when following the ketogenic diet as you don't want to become dehydrated. Furthermore, as the insulin level in the blood drops, it will make the kidneys excrete sodium, which will also contribute to urination.

Headaches and Brain Fog

 As you switch to the new diet plan, it may mean lesser calories for you than what your body was used to. Although the diet plan isn't devised to make one get fewer nutrients than are required to operate energetically, it can, however, cause headaches in some people. 2 of the 5 research participants reported that their head felt heavy.

Brain fog is also a symptom of undergoing dietary changes and adjusting to the new diet plan. Brain fog occurs due to low levels of minerals, which occur due to the loss of water in the beginning. When the body loses water, it also loses minerals such as potassium, magnesium, and salt, which contribute to feeling drowsy, and fatigued. All participants experienced loss of energy at the beginning, which was compensated by the intake of salt and adding potassium rich foods such as avocados, leafy greens, and dairy foods in the diet plan. A little deviation from the daily caloric intake will not cause a lot of problems, for example when taking extra salt in case of a headache, especially when you're adopting the diet for a long term.

Constipation

Constipation occurs due to magnesium deficit in the body, which is lost due to water loss. To avoid constipation participants were asked to take magnesium supplements, however, only 1 in 5 faced minor constipation.

Sugar Craving

It's natural to experience sugar cravings, and all the participants faced it. However, sugar cravings can be stopped or controlled naturally by going for a daily walk. It increases the level of dopamine in the brain- a neurotransmitter, which controls the mood and sugar cravings. Higher levels of dopamine results in reduced sugar cravings and better moods. Supplements that help control sugar craving include alpha lipoic acid, zinc, vitamin E, chromium GTF, and vitamin B complex. Only take after consulting your physician.

All these symptoms were experienced by participants for the first one week and maximum two after which they felt that their body has adjusted to the new diet and routine. They started to feel more energetic and fresh as they got used to the new diet plan and consequently started losing weight. Some of the participants also included exercise in their daily routine. None of the participants used to do any sort of exercise before but since starting the ketogenic diet, they adopted walking, running or treadmill and crunches to feel more enthusiastic about their weight and felt their attitude towards weight change.

It's true that when you indulge in positive actions for the sake of good health, it affects the mood positively especially when you start experiencing changes in your body for the better. All participants had visibly better moods until the end of the study than in the beginning as they experienced weight loss and the positive effects of the ketogenic diet. It is no wonder that adopting your body to a new routine or system is difficult but when you experience positive results, it becomes an inspiration to do so.

All the participants of this research study experienced significant weight loss and seemed happy to take the first step of adopting a new lifestyle in the form of the ketogenic diet. When you are at a healthy weight, you feel good about yourself and sometimes all a person needs is a positive push in the right direction. Losing weight isn't difficult and shouldn't be, but all it needs is some determination and inspiration. When you stop eating the carbs that your body was used to, naturally you start craving for the sugars. However, when you get past that stage, and your body becomes used to the new routine, almost all your sugar cravings subside and the ketogenic diet is one of the best ways to lose weight faster as all your sugar needs are eliminated by switching the body to the alternate energy system.

CHAPTER7: 5 TIPS TO PREPARE FOR "KETO SUCCESS"

So if you are impressed by the results of the research participants, you can achieve the same results as well but for that you first need to make a commitment to yourself to strictly following the tips and dietary restrictions I will shortly mention. Other than that know that you must absolutely not cheat while following the ketogenic diet because once you trigger your body into a different process of deriving energy, it is already hard on your body to make the shift. By cheating or taking high carb foods even occasionally can confuse your system and make it difficult for the body to shift to the ketones to derive its energy. It will continue to derive its energy from glucose and thus, your attempts will fail. While you may be thinking that you're doing a good job, in reality you won't be and will not experience fat loss as promised. Here are some tips to get started on your ketogenic diet for weight loss:

Tip #1- Take Less Than 20g Carbs in a Day

The whole idea of the ketogenic diet to lose weight is based on the fact that you have to limit your carbs in order to kick-start the process of the body to use the fats to derive energy. It is necessary that you keep your carb intake to 20g or less if, you want to experience success with your diet plan. Count each and every ounce of carb that you're having from the foods that you are eating and if you're following a diet plan make sure you stick to it.

Tip #2- Derive 65% of Your Calories from Fat

The calories that you take should majorly come from the fat source, as the second important fact of the diet is this: you have to increase your fat intake for the diet to work. When you increase your fat intake only then will you trigger the alternate process of deriving energy, thus leading to weight loss. The remaining calories should come from protein and carbs. To be precise 30% from proteins and 5% of carbs. This means the least amount of calories should come from carbohydrates.

Tip #3- Increase Water Intake

As mentioned in the symptoms that you will face initially when starting the ketogenic diet, water loss is natural and will occur as your body gets rid of the glucose from the muscles and liver. This also means you will be losing the essential minerals from your body so you must increase your water intake from the start in order to avoid dehydration.

Tip #4- Avoid Exercise Initially

If you already do not exercise, it is important that you mustn't take the imitative now when starting the diet. The reasoning is simple which is that the diet will already put enough strain on your body that you must avoid putting more of it now. At least for the first 2-3 weeks, avoid any kind of extra movement. In the initial phase you will automatically be feeling less energized and fatigued which can make exercise difficult, so don't even try.

Tip #5- Be Prepared

So the last tip has to do with preparation in every way. From mentally preparing yourself to physically making changes in your lifestyle to adopt the new diet, you must be prepared and ready to take this as a challenge and remain steadfast in your endeavor. It won't be an easy journey initially, but I promise you if that you get past two weeks of this diet, you are on the road to success.

It is easier to follow the diet when you have a seven-day plan in front you and you prepare the foods in advance and store them to quickly put your breakfast, lunch or dinner together. Just as the participants were made to do in this research. When you know beforehand what you have to take throughout the day, it becomes easier to be on the diet.

Food Intake Do's and Don't's

It can be difficult to understand initially what foods you must take in your diet when following a ketogenic diet plan and which foods to avoid. Here are simple do's and don't's of the foods that you must remember and which can help you put together your own ketogenic diet plan. However, make sure you that if you're making your own plan, you strictly calculate the caloric intake throughout the day that you will consume through different foods.

Food to Consume

Fats

The major food caloric intake on this diet is going to come through fats but you need to ensure that you're eating the right kinds of fat. While planning your fat intake make sure you maintain a healthy balance between omega 3 and omega 6 fats. You can derive a healthy source of omega 3 from eating wild tuna, salmon, shellfish, and trout.

You can also intake saturated and monounsaturated fats, as they are less inflammatory and more chemically stable. Foods in this category will include egg yolks, coconut oil, macadamia nuts, butter, and avocado.

Be careful and try to minimize your intake of hydrogenated fats as they are linked with higher chances of developing coronary heart disease. While frying any of the food items opt for non-hydrogenated lards, ghee, coconut oil or beef as they cause less oxidization of the oil and leaves more essential fatty acids for you to consume. Nut or seed based foods can be high in inflammatory omega 6s so keep your intake of walnuts, pine nuts, corn oil or sunflower oil to a minimum.

Foods that are preferred as a source of fats and oils include:

- Chicken fat
- Olive oil
- Coconut butter
- Red palm oil
- Ghee
- Avocado
- Beef tallow
- Macadamia nuts
- Peanut butter
- Butter
- Non-hydrogenated lard
- Mayonnaise
- Coconut oil

Proteins

When it comes to proteins, you should choose organic or grass-fed foods if you can since this minimizes bacteria and hormone intake. Foods that you should stock up on for your source of protein include:

Shellfish- you can have lobster, scallops, oysters, clams, mussels and squids.

Whole eggs- you can have your eggs deviled, boiled, scrambled, and poached for the best source of protein.

Fish- wild fish like cod, flounder, catfish, mackerel, salmon, trout, snapper and tuna is preferred.

Pork- there is added sugar in ham, but you can rely on pork chops and pork loin safely.

Poultry- you can have chicken, quail, duck or pheasant.

Meat- try to have grass fed meat of goat, lamb, beef or veal for a better count of fatty acids.

Peanut butter- peanut butter can have a high count of omega 6 and carbohydrates so be careful with its intake. Choose natural peanut butter and try having macadamia butter if possible.

Vegetables

You can have organic vegetables while on the ketogenic diet, but if you can't find organic ones, it's not that big a deal. Preferable vegetables include anything that grows above the ground. However, some vegetables are high in sugar and provide little nutritional benefit, so you want to make sure you stay clear of those. Focus on vegetables that are high in nutrients and low in carbohydrates, which would be dark and leafy vegetables such as spinach and kale.

Dairy Products

Choose full-fat raw or organic milk products while on the ketogenic diet to be successful. Avoid low-fat or fat-free products. These dairy products can include sour cream, hard and soft cheeses heavy whipping cream, and cottage cheese.

Nuts and Seeds

Our participants were allowed to have nuts and seeds as a snack and you can have them too. Make sure you roast whatever type of nuts you are eating to remove their anti-nutrients. One type of nuts to steer clear of on this diet are peanuts, being essentially legumes. Here are the other nuts and seeds you should stock on:

Cashews and pistachios: keep track of your intake of these as they are high in carbs

Macadamias, walnuts, and almonds: you can have them in small amounts as a snack as they are the best when it comes to the carb count.

Beverages

Dehydration is an effect that commonly accompanies the ketogenic diet, and if you are prone to bladder pain or urinary tract infections, then you must be adequately prepared beforehand to avoid any such problems. Make sure you are drinking the minimum 8 glasses of water, but if you need to drink more to stay hydrated, make sure you do. Apart from drinking plenty of water, you can have coffee or tea whichever you prefer, but in moderation because you may be taking sugar in your tea/coffee, and that's what you have to avoid.

What promotes success on a ketogenic diet is keeping your sugar cravings to a minimum level and taking sweeteners won't help achieve that. If you must rely on sweeteners, opt for liquid sweeteners that don't have added binders like maltodextrin or dextrose that have carbs.

Spices

While preparing any of your ketogenic food, you have to count in the spices as well as these have carbs in them. So a pinch of salt or black pepper is a pinch of carb as well; make sure you don't skip it while counting your calories. Pre-made spices usually have added sugars, so if you're purchasing any of these, make sure you carefully read the label. Table salt is usually mixed with powdered dextrose, so sea salt is the better choice. Other spices that you can count in and include in your foods are:

- Rosemary
- Cumin
- Basil
- Chili powder
- Black pepper
- Oregano
- Sage
- Parsley
- Cayenne pepper

- Turmeric
- Cilantro
- Cinnamon
- Thyme

Foods to Avoid On the Ketogenic Diet

In the section above, we have so far covered the foods that you should be focusing on if you want to achieve effective results with the ketogenic diet plan. Some foods are sneaky and not a good choice to include, even for a snack. Remember that you are trying to cut out the carbs from your diet to allow your body to derive its energy from an alternate source which is the ketones. Unless you don't limit your carbs to the minimum level, this will not become possible. Some foods to strictly avoid include:

- Avoid onion powder, allspice, bay leaves, cardamom, garlic powder and ginger as these have more carbs than any other spices.
- Avoid raspberries, cranberries and blueberries due to their high sugar content.
- Avoid tomato sauce and canned diced tomatoes as they have large amount of sugars in them
- Limit and eliminate if you can your intake of diet soda
- Flu remedies, cough syrups, and cold medication also contain carbs so ensure you are not taking them unnecessarily or for minimal influenza treatment. Watch out your dose intake as well if you take these syrups.

CHAPTER 8: YUMMY RECIPES

With all the food do's and don't's, it can get difficult to prepare your meals. It's very important to be well prepared before you embark on the ketogenic diet. Not just mentally but also with a recipe card in your hands and a meal plan that has your calories listed so that you know what you are eating and when. If you start your diet without a plan and without counting your calories, you won't know your daily caloric intake and whether you are keeping within the prescribed grams for fat, protein and carbohydrates.

Spending time to devise your meals beforehand, doing your pantry shopping accordingly will help you be fully prepared and in control of what you are eating. Any meals that you cook make sure you are aware of their caloric content and the amount of source of these calories.

To help you out, here are some recipes from the menu devised for our participants which you can use to prepare your own plan according to your preferences:

Sausage and Spinach Frittata

Ingredients:

- Sausage roll: 12 oz
- Frozen chopped spinach (thawed and drained): 10 oz
- Eggs: 12
- Crumbled Feta Cheese: ½ cup
- Heavy cream: ½ cup
- Salt: ½ tsp
- Ground nutmeg: ¼ tsp
- Black pepper: ¼ tsp
- Unsweetened plain almond milk: ½ cup

Preparation Method:

- Mix the raw sausage and spinach in a bowl breaking each into small pieces. Sprinkle the feta cheese and toss until combined. Spread the mixture on a greased casserole dish or in greased muffin cups.
- In another large bowl, beat the eggs, almond milk, pepper, cream and nutmeg and pour in the pan or muffin cups 3/4th of the way.
- Put the pan or muffin cups for baking at 375 degrees F. bake the muffin cups for 30 minutes and the casserole for 50 minutes. Make sure it is fully set before you take it out.
- Ready to serve at room temperature.

Yield: 12 squares or 18 muffin cups

Nutritional information per serving:

137 calories, 10g fat, 1g net carbs, 8g protein (muffins)

206 calories, 1.4g net carbs, 16g fat, 12g protein (squares)

Egg Salad
Ingredients:

- Eggs: 6
- Mayonnaise: 2 tbsp
- Dijon mustard: 1 tsp
- Lite Salt: ¼ tsp
- Lemon juice: 1 tsp
- Kosher salt and pepper: to taste

Preparation Method:

- Cover the eggs with cold water in a saucepan. Boil for ten minutes, take out and peel. Pulse the eggs in food processor until chopped.
- Mix in lemon juice, mustard, salt, pepper mayonnaise
- Add lettuce leaves or bacon when serving. (Optional)

Yield: Serves 4

Nutritional information per serving:

166 calories, 10g protein, 0.85g net carbs, 14g fat

Cauliflower gratin
Ingredients:

- Cauliflower florets: 4 cups
- Butter: 4 tbsp
- Heavy whipping cream: 1/3 cup
- Pepper jack cheese: 6 slices

- Salt and pepper: to taste

Preparation Method:

- Combine the butter, cauliflower, cream, salt and pepper. Mix thoroughly
- Put it on high in the microwave until its soft (approximately 25 minutes)
- Once it's soft, take it out and mash it adjusting the salt and pepper.
- Microwave for another 2 minutes with the cheese slices on top
- Serve and enjoy

Yield: Serves 6

Nutritional information per serving:

215 calories, 2g net carb, 6g protein, 19g fat.

Cream Cheese Pancakes

Ingredients:

- Cream cheese: 2 oz
- Eggs: 2
- Cinnamon: ½ tsp
- Sweetener: 1 packet

Preparation Method:

- Blend all ingredients until smooth. Let it rest for 2 minutes for the bubbles to subside
- Take a pan and grease with butter or pam spray. Put on heat and pour ¼ of the batter.
- Cook until golden, flip and cook for another 1 minute.
- Prepare more pancakes using the batter in the same way.
- Serve with sugar free syrup.

Yield: Serves 4

Nutritional information per serving:

344 calories, 2.5g carbohydrates, 17g protein, 29g fat.

Chili Spaghetti Squash

Ingredients:

(For chili)

- Lean ground beef: 1 lb
- Ground coriander: 1 tsp
- Ground Cumin: 1 tsp
- Garlic powder: ½ tsp

- Prepared salsa: ½ cup
- Dried oregano: 1 tsp
- Chopped chipotles: 1 tbsp (optional)

(For casserole)

- Cooked spaghetti squash: 4 cups
- Melted butter: 2 tbsp
- Chopped cilantro
- Sour cream: ¾ cup
- Shredded Mexican cheese: 1 ¾ cup

Preparation Method:

Prepare the chili:

- Brown the meat eat adding salt and pepper. Discard any extra fat and add chili ingredients.
- Leave to simmer for 10 minutes.

Prepare the casserole:

- Combine the spaghetti squash and butter in a bowl. Add salt and pepper to taste
- Take a casserole dish and spread out the squash. Sprinkle with shredded cheese. Layer the sour cream and chili. Finish topping with any remaining shredded cheese.
- Turn the oven to 350 degrees and let it bake for 30 minutes
- Serve with sour cream, salsa or cilantro.

Yield: Serves 8

Nutritional information per serving:

284 calories, 6g net carbs, 20g fat, 23g protein.

Anti-Pasta Salad

Ingredients:

- Chopped cauliflower: 2 cups
- Chopped radicchio: ½ cup
- Chopped artichoke hearts: ½ cup
- Grated parmesan: ½ cup
- Chopped basil: 1/3 cup
- Chopped sundried tomatoes: 3 tbsp
- Chopped Kalamata olives: 3 tbsp
- Minced garlic clove: 1
- Balsamic vinegar: 3 tbsp
- Extra virgin olive oil: 3 tbsp
- Salt and pepper to taste

Preparation Method:

- Heat the cauliflower in the microwave for 5 minutes
- Mix the basil, radicchio, parmesan, artichoke hearts, olives, sundried tomatoes, and garlic in a bowl.
- In another bowl, mix olive oil and vinegar and pour over salad
- Season with salt and pepper to serve
- Serve and enjoy

Yield: Serves 8

Nutritional information per serving:

102 calories, 4g net carbs, 3g protein, 8g fat

Feta and Sundried Tomato Meatballs

Ingredients:

- Ground turkey: 1 lb
- Crumbled feta cheese: ¼ cup
- Chopped sundried tomatoes: 5 oz
- Fresh thyme leaves: 1 tbs
- Egg: 1
- Almond flour: ¼ cup
- Garlic powder: ½ tsp
- Water: 2 tbs
- Olive oil

Preparation Method:

- Mix all ingredients together in a small bowl except olive oil.
- Heat the oil in a large saute pan and fry the meatballs until crisp and brown.
- Cook for 3-4 minutes on each side.
- Serve with marinara sauce.

Yield: 16 meatballs

Nutritional information per serving:

89 calories, 0.65 net carbs, 6g protein, and 8g fat

Cuban Pot Roast

Ingredients:

- Boneless chuck roast: 2.5-3 lb
- Canned chopped green chilies: ½ cup
- Salsa verde: ½ cup
- Dried onion flakes: 2 tbsp
- Diced tomatoes: 1 cup
- Garlic powder: 1 tsp
- Salt: 1 tsp
- Red and yellow peppers: ½ cup
- Ground cumin: 2 tbsp
- Ground coriander: 1 tbsp
- Dried oregano: 1 tsp
- Apple cider vinegar: 2 tbsp
- Black pepper: ½ tsp
- Chili powder: 1 tbsp

Preparation Method:

- Season the roast with salt and pepper generously.
- Sear in hot pan until browned
- Add salsa verde, tomatoes and chilis to the meat in pan.
- Bring to boil and pour the meat over in the crock pot.
- Stir in the onion flakes, salt, pepper, garlic, coriander, cumin, oregano, chili powder, black pepper, and apple cider vinegar.
- Cook on high heat for four hours and on low heat for 6 hours. Make sure the meat has become tender.
- Serve fresh.

Yield: Serves 10

Nutritional information per serving:

271 calories, 2g net carbs, 19g fat, 20g protein

CHAPTER 9: MY CONCLUSION

Starting any kind of diet requires determination and willingness. If you are overweight or obese and looking for a quick fix, understand that there is no such thing when it comes to losing weight. Your body is a complex machine running on multiple intricate mechanisms, and you should respect it. The ketogenic diet does help lose weight relatively faster because of the way it works. Sugars are bad for our health and the increased sugar intake already part of our lifestyle spells danger. The ketogenic diet limits these sugars and instead helps to trigger the ketones process from which our body can derive energy

Before conducting this research, I had my doubts about the ketogenic diet just like everyone else who thinks the low carb diets are yet another fad. But after having personally conducted this research with the help of two assistants, I was convinced that the diet is indeed helpful in losing weight. My personal take from this research which I would like to share with you all so that you may also benefit just as the participants in the study did, is to keep at it no matter what. Initially, following the ketogenic diet may seem difficult, and it will be, because you are in essence trying to make your body used to a new lifestyle and diet, but that is the case with all kinds of diets. Have a plan in place and prepare your menus in advance so that you don't find a chance to overeat or skin the keto diet once in a while. Know that any over-intake of carbs can prolong the effects of the diet as the adaptation process slows down.

Make a list of foods to eat and those to avoid and stick it on your refrigerator so that you don't forget. You can even print the menu plan from the book and use it to prepare your weekly plan. Just know what calories you are intaking when you plan to switch other foods in the plan. If you don't know what your daily carbohydrate, fat and protein intake then it's a waste to think that you're following the keto diet because maintaining the right levels of each are crucial to finding success on the keto diet.

Counting the carbs is an important part of the keto diet program, and you absolutely need to know how to do it properly. Get a carb counter guide if you feel that would help. It's also important to note there that before you get started you may have to clean sweep your entire kitchen. You can't let high carb foods lying around because it will be too difficult to avoid them then. Make sure you give away your unhealthy food choices before starting.

I met with the research participants every week to get an update on their progress and monitor their weight levels. We discussed different issues that the participants faced during the keto diet which I have mentioned above so that you may understand the initial symptoms of following this diet and which are normal. If you face any symptoms other than these, then it's important to see your physician before continuing on the new diet. Limit your exercise activity during the first few weeks of starting the diet because your body will already be feeling drained, and you don't want to put too much pressure on it in the starting. You may start exercising as well after 2-3 weeks have passed, and you have gotten into the new routine.

I wish you all the best for starting your journey on the road to a healthy lifestyle. It will not be easy, but I promise you that if you remain determined, you will get there, and with a bang at that! Focus on the end goal and if you include a friend or partner with you, following the keto diet plan can become easy. Be sure to check your progress and count your carbs for each meal. I have complete faith in you!